Pg. 36°
for sum
of why

The Turbo-Protein Diet

The author has developed and tested a remarkable diet based on the body's own metabolic principles. At last, significant weight loss can be achieved safely. At the same time, this diet defeats the tendency for rapid weight rebound. Unlike conventional fad diets, this scientific diet stimulates thyroid gland function so that more of the thyroid hormone called T_4 is created. This hormone is then converted into high quantities of the extremely metabolically-active T_3 hormone, which turns up the body's calorie burning furnace so well that no more fat can be stored.

Remarkable, safe weight loss can be achieved in only one to two weeks on this unique soy protein diet. Unlike other diets, with this diet the body does not simply eliminate water and muscle tissue—but actually burns fat. At the same time, the body is supplied with substances that protect it from "free radicals," molecules that can contribute to many "civilization diseases," everything from arteriosclerosis to polyarthritis.

Best of all, once the diet is completed, the body has been retrained. Reduced weight can be maintained without any difficulty; there is no tendency for the weight to bounce back—the notorious "yo-yo effect" is gone for good!

The Turbo-Protein Diet
Stop Yo-Yo Dieting Forever

The scientific European diet that takes off weight and trains the body to stay slender forever ...

Dieter Markert

BioMed International, L.P.
Houston, Texas

Copyright 1999, BioMed International, L.P.

All rights reserved. This book may not be duplicated in any way without the express written consent of the authors, except in the form of brief excerpts or quotations for the purposes of review. The information contained herein is for the personal use of the reader, and may not be incorporated in any commercial programs or other books, databases, or any kind of software without the written consent of the publisher or author. Making copies of this book, or any portion of it, for any purpose other than your own, is a violation of United States copyright laws.

Published by:
BioMed International, L.P.
3310 Richmond Ave., Ste. 100
Houston, TX 77098

ISBN: 0-9667285-1-3

Book Production: Phelps & Associates
Cover design: Knockout Design
Typography: Janice Phelps
Editor: Peter Bumpus
Illustrations: Matthias Wagner
Printer: United Graphics
PRINTED IN THE UNITED STATES OF AMERICA
Environmental note: All printed materials used in this paperback have been produced with environmental considerations in mind.

Cataloging-in-Publication Data
(Provided by Quality Books, Inc.)
Markert, Dieter, 1945-
    The turbo-protein diet : stop yo-yo dieting forever /
Dieter Markert. -- 1st ed.
    p. cm.
    Includes bibliographical references.
    Preassigned LCCN: 98-73951
    ISBN: 0-9667285-1-3

    1. Reducing diets. 2. High-protein diet. 3. Soy proteins
--Therapeutic use. I. Title.

RM222.2.M37 1998   613.2'5
                        QBI98-1339

TABLE OF CONTENTS

Readers are advised to consult a physician and undergo a thorough check-up before starting the diet and an accompanying exercise program.

People with cardiovascular, circulatory, or thyroid problems as well as diabetics, or those who must regularly take medication, should, as a matter of course, participate in a diet program only under a physician's watchful care.

The Turbo-Protein Diet is not intended to replace medical advice.

INTRODUCTION

I t's enough to drive you crazy! We live in a well-fed society of plenty where there is no major threat to our personal survival. Our supermarkets offer us countless delicacies from all over the world. Even pet food manufacturers have discovered gourmet tastes among the four-legged consumers and have come up with luxury food for pets.

We can stretch our legs contentedly in front of the television, snack on something sweet or fat and salty, and surf through entertaining programs without a care in the world. Slender models swing their way through endless advertisements: feather light, smooth-skinned, free of care. They advertise with provocative nonchalance for beer, chocolate bars, soft drinks.

Click. Talk show: With grave faces, a group of doctors declares that salvation is a thin waist.

Today, life's ideal line is the "Slim Line." Fat is mega-out. Every gram of fat appears suspicious, and anyway: Being overweight is ugly. The print media join this relentless chorus. Wherever one turns, the message is a constant barrage.

Trapped in this way, one's glance is naturally caught by an enticing ad that promises: Lose umpteen pounds in only one week! Nearby, an alluring blond beauty stretches in a tiny bikini. Lose a few pounds (of water) silly! So you think, okay, why not?

This is where things begin to get serious. There is an outrageous discrepancy between surplus abundance on the one hand, and the strict minimalism of the fragile Barbie-look on the other. This creates a powerful undertow that allows the most doubtful sort of "diet prophets" to suck in gullible victims and sometimes realize tremendous profits.

Last year for instance, 50 billion dollars were spent on diets in the U.S. alone. All these (wonder) diets have a decisive disadvantage: They cast an eye solely on the scales and disregard the body's biological laws and physiological needs. The physician is hopelessly overtaxed in the role as potential helper, consultant, and companion while attempting to help patients reach their ideal weights, because dietetics and nutrition physiology are not included in the normal study of medicine. Food chemists, psychologists, and pharmacists have taken the matter into their own hands—much to the detriment of those affected, as we shall see.

Assume that Ms. "X" decided to go on a fad diet and managed to stick with it. When she is finished and returns to the world of the Normal Eater, two things become apparent to her: First, she is plagued by periods of voracious appetite, and second, she stuffs herself. She suffers from a feeling of inner emptiness and cannot help but try to fill this hole; soon she has regained her former weight. And what's worse, she gained weight faster than before her diet. What should she do? For her, the matter is clear—another diet!

In this way, diet fads are spontaneously generated, and rapid weight rebound, the "yo-yo effect," sets in all on its own. Ultimately, adversity of the worst sort threatens Ms. X: chronic high blood sugar with increased insulin production, high blood pressure, arteriosclerosis, and diabetes mellitus—the "metabolic syndrome."

In Europe and North America, the world's oases of surplus, hundreds of people die every year from improper and unhealthy diet programs. Again and again the fact is ignored that the body needs certain basic substances during a time of nourishment reduction. Without these substances, the body cannot function. When the body doesn't receive the vital proteins it needs in precisely balanced amounts, as is commonly the case in most weight-reduction programs, serious to acute damage to health is a real threat—from cardiac irregularities to heart attacks to collapse of the immune system. I myself have witnessed death from meningitis caused by weakness in the body's defense mechanisms resulting from a person's diet. The victim: a well-known German executive. The culprit: one of the many "wonder diets," which can be freely bought practically everywhere.

So why another new diet?

This diet is both healthy and effective—and it circumnavigates the dangerous cliffs and reefs the human body has set up, for good reason, around the "Blissful Island of the Ideal Weight." The Turbo-Protein Diet is very easy to apply, as you will soon see. Supported by a few exercise routines and some sports, this diet is extremely powerful. It is not some sort of new "wonder" diet, however. The Turbo-Protein Diet's phenomenal success is based on the fact that it respects and uses the body's own physiological laws and processes to achieve a healthy reduction in weight.

In the theoretical portion of this book, these laws and processes will be explained. I want to describe the decisive difference between a typical wonder diet and my revolutionary, well-tested protein diet. Among other things, you will learn about the vital processes involved in cell metabolism and how a well-regulated metabolism can maintain a slender profile and ward off disease.

For instance, you will learn about the harmful free radicals and what they have to do with the yo-yo effect of weight gain and loss, and how you can avoid or resist this reaction effectively. A relatively detailed historical study will make it clear to you how nourishment, health, and survival have evolved over the course of human development, and how our bodies unshakably follow these same natural laws to this day.

In principle, it is not necessary to understand the underlying medical and physiological laws to effectively apply the Turbo-Protein Diet. Hence, you can turn to the book's second section and begin the diet program at once. Later, you can go back and convince yourself that you are on the right track by reading the first section.

The diet provides you with three gifts:
- A slender, robust figure, without leaching out the body or making it sick,
- Improved quality of life,
- Increased energy and vigor.

I wish you success and satisfaction in reducing your weight with this diet!

—Dieter Markert

Part One
The Basics

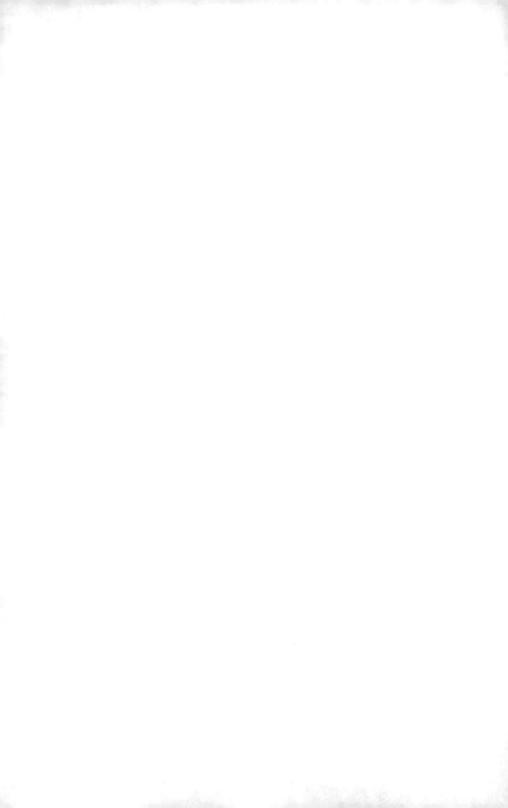

THE BODY'S SURVIVAL STRATEGIES

Some 3.5 million years ago, when Lucy, the best known primitive woman, was wandering through what is now Ethiopia, her clan's agriculture was still very undeveloped. Collecting food and struggling to survive dominated her daily existence.

The presence of only a few sharp, fang-like teeth in early humans such as Lucy indicate that although our forebears were omnivores (who eat both plants and animals), they mostly consumed plants. In order to get enough to eat and to sufficiently sustain their bodily functions for reproduction, these primitive clans would have had to consume a fairly large amount of fruits, roots, insects, and small animals. Therefore they must have spent the entire day searching for and collecting edible food.

But when the hunter–gatherers appeared on the scene about 2.5 million years ago, the situation changed dramatically. Hunted animals provided proteins—amino acid compounds in concentrated form—which are the vital building blocks of human life. Suddenly, humans were freed from the burden of constantly gathering food to survive. Now, they had time to create new and improved tools. During this developmental thrust forward, human posture became more upright, the skull expanded, and the cerebrum developed enormously. *Homo erectus* is born, distinct from its pre-hominid forefathers.

At exactly the same time, humans also developed the great principle of survival, which has yet to lose its effectiveness—the fight or flight response. For example, let's assume that Lucy is surprised by an enemy while she is gathering fruits and nuts. In order to survive, she must recognize the danger and instantly do one of two things: If she is lucky, she can flee; if not, she must fight for her life. In primitive times, the threat could have been a predatory beast; nowadays it could be the boss at work, but in either case, the human survival response unfolds in the same way —fright, stress, and massive release of stress hormones. The flight reflex leads to an immediate drainage of the energy supply, which is principally the glucose reserves in the muscle tissue and liver. In lesser amounts, fatty acids are also made available from the fatty tissue. Note however: These fatty acids belong to the body's permanent reserve and are eminently important for survival. That is why the body stores them to be transformed into energy, and that is why they are mobilized during stress situations. This fat is stored in many areas of the body and is partly responsible for the grotesque distribution of fat—a phenomenon that is one of the major evils resulting from many of today's fad diets.

The flight was successful—Lucy is safe. Now she can replenish her glucose reserves by eating. If there's nothing to eat, her body will create sugar for energy by breaking down bodily protein, chiefly from muscle tissue. Ever since the earliest times, human populations have been decimated by terrible droughts, bad harvests, plagues, and epidemics. Without emergency strategies for coping, humans would have died out long ago. In addition to creating energy reserves, humans also developed a second aid to survival: the adipostat, a control center in the interbrain (diencephalon) that helps regulate metabolism and feelings of hunger and satiation.

Many ages ago, early man had to live with the fact that sometimes there was a surplus of food available, and at other times there were very limited sources of nourishment, or none at all. In times of plenty, everyone filled their belly as full as possible. To prepare for bad times, the body stored up more than enough fat in its depots. More than enough carbohydrate was converted to reserve fat as well. hell-ooo !

For instance, let's assume our foremother Lucy had a fat percentage that gave her 65 pounds of fat by weight. One pound of pure fat tissue has a caloric value of about 2,750 calories. Considering a basic requirement of 2,000 calories per day, and assuming that Lucy can find a handful of nuts, berries, and a bit of wild oats here and there, she could easily survive and manage to assure her child's survival for about a half a year on a lean diet.

Once the fat reserves have been used up and a sudden time of plenty begins, Lucy has to make sure that she rebuilds her padding of excess fat as fast as possible. The adipostat controls this process—it is the most important guarantee for preservation of the species. This survival controller par excellence is found in the interbrain next to the thermoregulation center and functions by a feedback mechanism where sensors (leptin hormones) report the current level of fat reserves to the adipostat. These hormones know what to report based on the insulin level. In times of need, if Lucy loses a considerable amount of her fat padding, her adipostat is put into a state of constant alarm by mobilized fatty acids, freed leptins (the sensors), and a barrage of stress hormones. In other words, Lucy is plagued by acute attacks of hunger.

At the same time, Lucy's thyroid gland reduces her metabolic rate in order to save as much energy as possible. So Lucy can think of nothing besides eat, eat, eat. Her body's metabolism drops to save, save, save energy. Lucy pursues food relentlessly, until she manages to put on a sufficient layer of fat. Only when the body's target fat level has been reached does her adipostat give her any peace. Thanks to the lower metabolism, fat storage has occurred in only half the time. Moreover, the body notes its successful fat-storing strategy for the next time there is a reduction in intake. Today, this primitive physiological survival strategy creates the dreaded yo-yo effect of rapid weight gain after a typical fad diet. Anyone who has tried a conventional diet can confirm this process.

NOURISHMENT
IN HUMAN HISTORY

L et's jump from the earliest human epoch to the Middle
Ages and take a look at how eating habits changed over
the centuries.

Meats—especially the fatty pieces—were soon the main
focus for meals in princely courts as well as at farmers' feasts. Up
until the end of the Middle Ages, honey was the most important
sweetener. Processed or "table" sugar, on the other hand, was a
great rarity until the 15th century and was predominantly used as
medicine.

Salt played a great role in the economy, especially in
central Europe. It was extremely important not only as a spice
and taste enhancer, but as the most common preservative for
meat and fish.

Bread, especially white bread, was a basic food of the better
classes, including priests and monks. For most people, who were
farmers, bread did not play a large role at the time. Their food staples were mashed cereals and grain gruel along with the most
important component, legumes.

Table fruit was considered a luxury. The cultivation of fruit
was primarily promoted in cloisters and then spread to peasants'
farm gardens. In some regions, fruit wines made from very sour
apples and pears had been a traditional drink since the Middle

Ages. Beer had a role in folk nutrition that is hardly imaginable today: In the 17th century, breakfast often consisted of beer soup. These beer soups were widespread in some parts of Germany until the end of the 18th century.

The potato deserves special notice, since it had a hard time being accepted as folk nourishment. Potatoes were widespread in Ireland and England by the 17th century, and from there reached Germany along the lower Rhine and in Palatine. The Palatines brought the potato to Brandenburg, but it was the famines of the late 18th and early 19th centuries that made the potato a German staple.

These examples illustrate that human eating habits change over time, and that physiological requirements may be overwhelmed by cultural preferences. A closer look would show that harvest yields and population densities were always crucial in determining how people ate as well. Now, let's take another jump to further examine the Middle Ages....

In the second half of the 14th century, bad harvests and scourging epidemics decimated a third to a fourth of the population of Europe. The result was a shortage of workers, which led to an increase in wages, which in turn had a lasting effect on the lifestyle (diet) of the working population. Among other things, a considerable increase in meat consumption occurred; around the year 1400 it is estimated that an average of 220 pounds of meat were eaten per person per year. That's about 25 percent higher than today.

By the end of the 15th century however, the long stagnant population started to grow. Between 1470 and 1620, the population of central Europe grew by approximately 60 percent. Around

1800, and despite terrible losses due to the Thirty Years' War, the population within the boundaries of what later was the German Reich reached a temporary all-time high of about 24 million people. At this point the land's ability to produce enough food was exhausted. Whatever grazing land could be plowed under was planted in crops. Nevertheless, yields fell due to a lack of fertilizer.

The food situation remained very strained in the 18th and 19th centuries. One bad harvest followed another, resulting in serious famines. But scientific discoveries in the 18th century made possible by the Age of Enlightenment, combined with the more permissive atmosphere of liberalism, created the Industrial Revolution in England by the middle of the 18th century. At first the new achievements had a devastating impact. The mechanization of production destroyed jobs. Improved overseas shipping and newly developed methods of preservation resulted in a fall in agricultural prices and drove large numbers of small farmers into the cities in search of a better life. Medical progress reduced the death rate and sped up population growth. The result was mass unemployment, declining wages, and the spread of slums in the developing big industrial cities.

Finally, scientific and technical progress brought about a balance. A series of hunger catastrophes between 1845 and 1848 became the last in the Western world that were not triggered by war. Increased productivity from increased mechanization led to a shift in wealth, which allowed for a decrease in working hours, and within a few decades the beginnings of a social security system. Scientific discoveries including new fertilizers and high-yield, more disease-resistant grains and domestic animal breeds helped distribute basic foodstuffs and reduce food prices to an unexpected extent. Also, longer life expectancy did not bring about increased population growth in Europe. Instead, increased education throughout the population led to self-limiting birth control that adjusted to economic conditions.

This impressive development can be followed by studying the consumption data provided by agrarian statistics, which despite certain uncertainties allow one to trace back to the middle of the 19th century with considerable accuracy. After 1850 a strong rise in the consumption of bread, grains, and potatoes satisfied the need for basic staple foods to stave off hunger. By the end of the century, the provision of staples covered the needs of the population. Since then, the consumption of bread grains (particularly rye) and potatoes has fallen sharply. Today, we note a rise in grain consumption that can be attributed to the success of the campaign for a more balanced diet. On the other hand, the decline in consumption of the less liked but filling legumes can be explained as a result of rising meat and fat consumption.

Several factors caused progressively increasing sugar consumption since 1850. The first, naturally, is the appetite for something sweet. But the phenomenon is mostly due to the successful cultivation of sugar-rich beets, which allowed sweets and sugar to become widely available to all sections of the population at affordable prices.

Fresh fruit was a luxury item even by the middle of the 19th century. Because fresh fruit is highly perishable, middle-class households generally kept dried fruits to refine their menus. Farm workers and artisans in south Germany consumed large quantities of thin fruit ciders as a refreshing drink. A turning point was the introduction of tree nurseries from England, which led to cultivation of fruit varieties that stored better and to the planting of extensive fruit orchards. Fruit cultivation caught on quickly, largely due to the huge grain imports from the United States after the end of the Civil War, which sharply lowered grain prices. The local agricultural economy was spurred to switch to more competitive products, advancing fruit cultivation as well as production of sugar beets and potatoes. Since the purchasing power of the population rose at the same time, fruit quickly became cheaper and more popular. The striking increase in fruit consumption since World War II is largely due to the great progress made in fruit preservation and storage, making fruit consumption almost independent of the season.

In the case of vegetables, consumption patterns underwent a fundamental change only after World War II. Up until then, large vegetables such as cabbage, carrots, cucumbers, and onions—in North Germany beets and kale as well—appeared on tables. The finer sorts of vegetables which now dominate the market, especially tomatoes and lettuces, but also cauliflower, brussels sprouts, and green beans, were up to that time considered gourmet items reserved for special occasions.

Cheese consumption boomed after World War II, reaching the pre-war level in 1952, increasing by over twice that amount since then. The consumption of meat rose particularly fast. The pre-war level was attained between 1956 and 1957. Afterwards beef consumption rose by a third, pork consumption doubled, and fowl consumption quadrupled!

The consumption of meat fat runs parallel to meat consumption only until the turn of the century. Afterwards the less-favored fats, especially beef tallow, were apparently no longer desired and instead were used in industry for soap, candles, and so forth. It is hard to estimate how much was processed into sausage meat, however. On the other hand, the consumption of vegetable oils has risen since the turn of the century. They played an important role, particularly fats based on coconut oil, between the world wars. After World War II, the proportion of other vegetable oils rose. Now they account for 40 percent of all vegetable fats, including margarine.

Surprisingly, the data derived from agrarian statistics shows that the consumption of food energy has barely changed since the supply bottlenecks before the turn of the century. The proportion of protein in the diet was reduced only during times of emergency or crisis; in times of normal or lavish food supply, it remained fairly constant averaging 85 to 95 grams a day, in exceptional cases, 100 grams. The proportion of fat in energy consumption, on the other hand, has risen sharply: from only a bit more than 20 percent around 1850 to about 27 percent before World War I, with a present level at almost 40 percent. Accordingly, the proportion of carbohydrates in the diet has fallen.

And finally, here are a few statistics on the development of alcohol consumption. Alcohol has always played a role in human nutritional intake. We have more exact (German) statistics since 1888. These reveal that in 1888 the per capita annual consumption of brandy and whiskey was 4 gallons, and for beer the average was 30 gallons a year. Wine consumption was identified only after 1898, with 2.1 gallons a year, which is very low. Alcohol consumption sank sharply between the two World Wars (from 1935 to 1938: 0.9 gallons of brandy; 1.9 gallons of wine; 18 gallons of beer per person per year). A gradual rise after World

War II took place mainly in beer and wine consumption; brandy consumption only rose temporarily (from 1979 to 1982: 1.5 gallons of brandy; 7.2 gallons of wine; 42.2 gallons of beer per person per year). Hence, we have again reached the average level of consumption as before the turn of the century: about 26 grams of alcohol per person every day. A small comfort may be found in the fact that in those days almost 50 percent of alcohol consumption was in hard drinks, whereas now these make up only 20 percent of alcohol intake.

This historical review challenges us to define our current situation in comparison to the past. With the help of these loosely drawn main lines of development, we can venture the following:

Until the last third of the 19th century, life in central and northern Europe was primarily dominated by periods in which population masses had to live with barely more than the minimum required food, and for longer periods they had to survive on less than the minimum—which, remember, is acceptable (and possibly preferable) from the evolutionary standpoint. We know that the population as a whole succeeded in adjusting to these meager living conditions, even in the face of daily hard physical labor, because the population increased considerably during this time. True, the population density was repeatedly cut down, but only by famines, epidemics, or wars, and the following generations always faced better living conditions and were able to make up the loss.

For a long time, scanty food supply acted as a population regulator. But as a result of the scientific and technical revolution, agriculture started to produce surplus food with considerably less human labor. In general, surplus food led to the consumption of excess fat, excess carbohydrates, and processed sugar, all in the presence of high alcohol intake. This development occurred within a very short time span, but a human physiological adjustment could not evolve so quickly. As a result, we now find ourselves in an "adjustment crisis," and therefore we must carefully consider our current diet with a fresh outlook. We must take sensible measures to shorten or terminate this crisis, in order to fight against its undesirable, indeed seriously threatening, consequences for our health.

This is the typical dilemma in all modern, Western, industrial nations: On the one hand, we have to limit our food intake to match our reduced energy requirements that are the result of the huge increase in automation in our professional lives, travel, and recreation. On the other hand, our requirement for essential nutrients has not lessened; in fact, often it has increased from chronic consumption of medication. Therefore, we can free ourselves from our adjustment crisis only by consuming the same amount of vital proteins, vitamins, and minerals, in less food.

Summation of current healthy dietary crisis

FOOD AND HEALTH

In almost all ancient religions, food was considered a gift from a benevolent old mother goddess figure, portrayed in hard times with a resentful character, the object of numerous sacred rites. Today the idea of food has been transformed. Without transition and incomprehensibly for most of us, food has become a sober mixture of chemical substances, often modified by chemical intervention.

How such a profound change (away from the natural balance of foods) could take place—during the Romantic Age no less—without incurring a backlash of some sort, is obvious. Opposing trends, however, followed in the footsteps of industrialization (with a time lag). They began in the first decades of the 19th century as vegetarianism in England and then spread to central Europe between 1867 (E. Baltzer) and the turn of the century (R. Steiner, M. Bircher-Benner). We don't want to attempt to describe these ideologically-based nutritional teachings, or to try to come to terms with such currently popular quality labels such as "biological" (used mostly in Europe) or "holistic." Instead, I would much rather explain the influence of nutrition on the healthy organism from a scientific point of view.

Nature has provided us with well-functioning systems to control our food and liquid intake. Hunger and thirst make it very clear to us when we need food or liquid, and the sense of repletion lets us know when our needs have been fulfilled. After a lavish meal we are flooded with a comfortable feeling, as are all beasts of prey, telling us our body has received enough to maintain functioning—we should now devote ourselves to getting some rest. Even our pets play or sleep only when they have full stomachs. All of this is controlled by centers in the brain stem that are easy to locate and that lie anatomically near each other.

A keen appetite for some particularly tasty morsel, coupled with a desire for variety, provides us with a regulatory mechanism that helps keep us from suffering specific nutrient deficiencies and protects our bodies from a glut of inappropriate nourishment. This mechanism is not—or at least is no longer—a reliable one, however. For example, if small children were allowed to consume food only according to their taste, the resulting nourishment would most probably not cover their bodily needs. Likewise, the odd cravings for certain kinds of food common during early pregnancy cannot be explained physiologically in terms of nutritional value.

Human food is generally made up of very complex chemical substances. It is not particularly surprising, therefore, that some types trigger side effects when consumed in extremely high dosages. Usually these are harmful side effects, for example with Vitamin A or Vitamin D poisoning, or the toxic effects of the essential mineral substances sodium, zinc, copper, and iron. The fact that harmful side effects are not found with all forms of nourishment is based on special protective mechanisms of the body that prevent excessive intake:

• Limited absorption capacity of the intestinal membrane,
• Hastened elimination through the urine or gall bladder

when concentration limits are exceeded, and

⟶ • Storage of surpluses in depots (especially in the liver, fatty tissue, and skeleton), which can be drawn upon in times of need.

Many of these modes of operation and their interconnections have not yet been comprehensively analyzed, since the ability of the human body to store essential nutrients greatly impedes experimental research in this particular area. A prerequisite for such research would require a test subject to voluntarily partake of an extremely limited, narrow diet in order to empty all the nutritional storage areas. Once this had taken place, one could begin to determine the requirements for specific nutrients by adding them to the diet and noting specific reactions. A series of such experiments was begun during World War II in the U.S. and England, but today no ethics commission would ever permit such work to be carried out.

Therefore it is clear that the relationship between nourishment and health cannot be definitively proven by means of purely scientific methods. On the other hand, it makes sense to consider the connection between nourishment and health disorders. But even here the researcher must work with complex chains of causalities with long-term consequences, which often conceal the real connection between cause and effect.

Health statistics in the Federal Republic of Germany illustrate how a sweeping change has taken place within only a few years—from a war economy with extremely scarce supplies to a surplus society of plenty. Since 1952, the first year in which unified, systematic cause-of-death statistics were carried out in Germany, there has been a drastic increase in the number of deaths due to coronary diseases, arterial circulatory disorders of the brain (both of these disorders are largely caused by arteriosclerosis), as well as due to diabetes mellitus, more or less critical fat metabolism disorders, and liver cirrhosis. West Germany rapidly developed a surplus of civilization illnesses, which had been observed in the United States for some time already. In America, intensive study had already begun regarding the causes of such diseases and the possibilities of counteracting them.

CARDIOVASCULAR DISEASES
AND THEIR CAUSES

Research concerning the causes of arteriosclerosis has always dominated the study of cardiovascular diseases. It was intensified after vascular diseases were discovered in the bodies of a considerable number of young American soldiers killed in Korea, and later in Vietnam. Soon afterwards the general public was informed that such diseases were not only common in high-stress executives, but had practically become a threatening folk epidemic. Since then, the death rate from heart disease for men in U.S. has fallen almost 30 percent. In contrast, the German death rate for such diseases has risen by more than 30 percent (in fact, for the age group 65 to 74, almost 60 percent). The total picture reveals that the German statistics for vascular disease have now nearly approached those in America.

From the beginning, it was understood that there are diverse causes for cardiovascular disease. It was assumed that too little exercise and too much food played an important role, although this was hard to prove definitively. It was particularly difficult to prove which nutritional factors were of critical importance for the formation of arteriosclerosis. On the other hand, proof that increased nicotine consumption contributed directly to the danger of a heart attack was rather quickly and unambiguously produced.

Over time, a large number of studies became available that substantiated important correlations between eating habits and arteriosclerosis. Furthermore, it has been proven that a drop in the serum cholesterol concentration in the blood reduces the risk of a heart attack, and that arteriosclerotic vascular changes can recede when there is a lasting reduction of high blood fat values. To achieve this, it is essential to bring about a consistent readjustment of life habits: quitting smoking, losing excess body weight until values are within the range of the Body Mass Index (see the table on page 28), reducing consumption of fats and salt, increasing intake of roughage, and the sensible increase of bodily activity.

Undeniably, there are people who simply possess a high natural resistance to arteriosclerosis, and others who suffer heart attacks or critical brain arteriosclerosis despite the fact that they have always pursued healthy living habits. Indeed, an inherited tendency to develop arteriosclerosis could be proven, although it seldom occurs. Far more likely, the very rapid increase of this disease has its explanation in the realities of how we live in a modern industrial society. Medical research has accepted the challenge, and in numerous countries around the world scientists are now trying to isolate the causes, processes, and possible preventive measures and treatments for arteriosclerosis.

Intensive research has evaluated increased levels of cholesterol and triglyceride (a fatty acid) in the blood. The important factor is the difference between low density serum cholesterol (LDL and VLDL) and high density (HDL). High levels of LDL and VLDL cholesterol are considered risk factors. When there is a surplus of molecules called "free radicals" in the blood as well, high levels of LDL and VLDL cholesterol can oxidize these particles and initiate a reaction that is fundamental to the formation of arteriosclerosis, and can lead to the congestion of arteries and the triggering of a heart attack or stroke.

In contrast, HDL cholesterol is the form in which cholesterol is transported to the liver. Higher concentrations of HDL cholesterol indicate that cholesterol is being broken down in the tissues, and thus there is a reduced risk of arteriosclerosis. A marked characteristic of this eminently vascular-protective HDL cholesterol is that its levels increase during times of hard physical labor or sports activity, thus becoming an inner shield against arteriosclerosis. Red wine, consumed moderately, apparently also has this effect, in somewhat weakened form.

It is very probable that increased concentrations of triglycerides in the blood can also be considered a risk factor, especially when larger amounts of fat are transferred from the liver to exterior tissue, which first and foremost happens after profuse carbohydrate-rich meals and heavy alcohol consumption. Decomposition products, which remain in the bloodstream after triglyceride has been passed on to the fat depot, further the formation of LDL cholesterol and tend to be stored in the blood vessels or oxidized via free radicals.

This brief overview should make it clear that lack of bodily exercise and bad eating habits cannot be separated from each other. Both play an important role in the development of what are in reality civilization diseases, which all together constitute a metabolic syndrome.

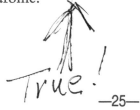

HOW DO I DETERMINE
MY NORMAL WEIGHT?

Today, "health" can be measured by considering body weight and other measurable risk factors. But in fact, the greater the excess weight, the more often other risk factors are present. The correlation between health and weight is not so simple however. In general, moderately overweight people need to reckon with only a few of these health risks. On the other hand, some people of ideal weight may be at risk for one or more of the typical civilization diseases. (This is particularly true for those who have high serum cholesterol levels caused by a genetic disposition.) For most people however—the risk of suffering from any aspect of the metabolic syndrome is practically zero if one engages in sports or other vigorous activity several times a week, eats healthy foods, and maintains a normal weight.

Normal weight? How do I know what is normal?

The once universal Broca formula used in Europe is outdated. This formula figures normal weight in kilos, by subtracting 100 from body height in centimeters. Unfortunately, the Broca method recommends weights that are too low for short people, and too high for tall ones. Similar weight-to-height tables were used by physicians in the U.S. The Body Mass Index (BMI) provides a much clearer picture of whether someone is over- or underweight.

1. Here is the formula:

$$BMI = \frac{703 \times Weight\ in\ Pounds}{Height\ in\ Inches \times Height\ in\ Inches}$$

2. The following standard values apply to adult men and women:

Within the limits of 20 to 25 for men and 19 to 24 for women, less disease and a lower death rate are observed (especially for values in the lower range of the norm). But the most important thing to remember is—don't worry about the cosmetic values of the numbers; instead, aim for a sense of well-being. Define your "dream" weight as the range within the norm where you feel good and are most productive.

For example: in most cases, men with values over 25 and women with over 24 are overweight, but competitive athletes and bodybuilders are an exception. Due to their powerful (and heavy) muscle packages, they can be very healthy with a higher BMI.

3. Representative statistics:

In 1978, for the first time, West Germany produced representative statistics describing the risks of being overweight. According to these figures, 5.5 percent of the men and 9 percent of the women over 18 were very overweight, and 35 percent of the men and 33 percent of the women were moderately overweight. The frequency of being overweight is not age-dependent. It is, however, clearly dependent on education and professional training. The higher the professional qualifications, the less chance of being overweight.

The share of young people between 18 to 34 years old was 14 percent in 1978—a considerable percentage. A further rise measured in 1982 and 1983 among children and young people confirmed these numbers. Among teenagers, on the other hand, a growing portion were underweight, with girls clearly in the majority. A survey revealed that a large number of these girls were consciously refraining from eating due to a fear of getting fat.

The number of underweight young girls has increased considerably since that time. They are usually the daughters of very slender mothers. It's apparent that we are running the danger of falling from one extreme into the other, and appropriate information should be used to stave off the dangerous effects of undernourishment as early as possible. The danger for young women is particularly severe when their energy and nutrient reserves are taxed considerably during pregnancy and lactation, since not only the mother is affected, but also the infant. A physician taking a critical look at the thin creatures who dominate fashion and lifestyle magazines—who are role models for girls and young women—is in for a grave shock. These magazine divas very likely suffer from serious hormone disturbances, most likely including the absence of menstrual periods. Their metabolism has probably shifted from the healthy build-up phase (anabolic) to the break-down (catabolic) phase, which normally occurs only during serious illness. It is a good bet that not one of these models could sprint to a bus or taxi without becoming totally exhausted. Nevertheless the girls of the world eagerly contend to imitate them.

Another cause of concern is the relatively high number of overweight children, both toddlers and schoolchildren. Undoubtedly health considerations on the part of the mother play a decisive role here. Enlightening these women about the vital importance of attending to certain lower limits of food intake certainly has more chance of success than a similar appeal to teenagers.

The need for an easily comprehensible definition of a healthy target weight for people of all ages and sizes—with both upper and lower limits for intervention—is obvious. The chart on page 32 offers you just this, based on the Body Mass Index.

4. Ideal body weight:

Attempting to use a theoretical "ideal" body weight as the only relevant measurement to indicate that the body has misdirected its allocation of energy resources (too much or too little fat) is never satisfactory for three reasons:

- It disregards different body builds,
- Weight fluctuates daily as fluid content in the body tissue changes, and
- It gives the wrong picture for people with well-developed muscles.

Measuring the thickness of hypodermic fatty tissue in the upper arm, hip, and on the front of the thigh provides a more reliable reading of the body's fat reserves. This can be done with special forceps or by ultrasound, and the result should be between 11 to 22 pounds, even for slender people.

Despite its inadequacies, checking weight is still favored in practice. Its invaluable advantage is that everyone can easily do it all by themselves. In addition, close observation of energy reserve factors can make up for the blurry definitions that weight by itself offers for assessing health.

Body Weight Table

Adult weight, with tolerance range figured according to height
(calculated by Body Mass Index)

Height	Weight in pounds	
	Men	Women
4'8"	–	100 (87–110)
4'9"	–	103 (89–112)
4'10"	–	106 (91–115)
4'11"	–	109 (93–119)
5'	122 (105–131)	112 (97–120)
5'1"	125 (107–134)	117 (101–129)
5'2"	129 (111–138)	121 (127–132)
5'3"	132 (112–141)	124 (107–135)
5'4"	135 (116–144)	127 (110–132)
5'5"	143 (121–153)	133 (116–145)
5'6"	146 (124–155)	136 (118–149)
5'7"	150 (128–160)	143 (121–153)
5'8"	153 (130–163)	143 (123–156)
5'9"	160 (136–171)	150 (130–164)
5'10"	164 (140–174)	153 (132–167)
5'11"	167 (143–178)	157 (135–172)
6'	171 (145–183)	161 (139–175)
6'1"	179 (152–190)	167 (144–183)
6'2"	182 (155–195)	–
6'3"	187 (158–199)	–
6'4"	195 (166–207)	–
6'5"	199 (169–211)	–

Body Mass Index:
Men: 23.5 (20–25)
Women: 22 (19–24)

THE ENERGY CARRIERS:
FATS AND CARBOHYDRATES

A s we have already discussed, fat ingestion has risen considerably faster than our total energy consumption. In the process, the chemical composition of consumed fats has shifted somewhat toward multiple unsaturated fatty acids. As a result of the increase in the portion of animal foods in our diet—largely due to the hidden fats in meats—there was a simultaneous rise in average cholesterol consumption. The high level of alcohol consumption has also had a damaging effect on the body's fat environment since the natural breakdown of alcohol creates the basic components required for increased fat synthesis.

In view of these tendencies we should always keep in mind that reducing our fat intake is one of the most important measures for preventing and fighting arteriosclerosis. The medical world's appeal to limit fat consumption recently received important support. Numerous studies have shown that the high level of fat in the diet of the populace of wealthy nations contributes considerably to the frequency of intestinal and breast cancer.

For people with higher energy requirements such as those who do hard physical labor or who compete in athletics, dietary fat can't be limited to the prescribed 30 percent of total calories if they want to maintain peak productivity. Assuming a normal blood-fat status, measuring dietary fat is not important for highly active people, since they have only a very minimal risk of suffering from arteriosclerosis. On the other hand however, people previously engaged in hard physical labor or athletics are in great danger if they suddenly retire from these activities, or are forced to make a break due to an accident. In these cases, careful supervision of diet and long-term medical treatment is absolutely necessary. Furthermore, as we shall see (see page 46), one must be somewhat active to maintain the function of glucose transport receptors, which allow glucose to be burned, and not stored as fat.

The human preference for fat in the diet is no accident. Fat improves the taste of food. Hence it is difficult to produce a low-fat sausage or cheese that will appeal to consumers. Furthermore, because fats stay in the stomach longer, they cause a longer sense of satiation. Thus, numerous calorie-reduced foods that have been created by reducing the level of fat have had little chance of long-term success, since the feeling of hunger returns soon after they have been consumed.

As far as quantity goes, carbohydrates are the most important energy carriers in our food. They must not be neglected in any discussion of overeating. The brief historical overview about human eating habits has already shown that the spectrum of carbohydrate-rich foods has changed considerably during the last hundred years. Above all, the share of energy-providing carbohydrates from foods such as potatoes and unpolished rice (high-molecular carbohydrates) has been continuously sinking, whereas the consumption of saccharose (cane and beet sugar) has been rising a lot. This has fundamentally changed carbohydrate metabolism.

Humans digest carbohydrates (also called starches) by splitting them into maltose (malt sugar) and maltotriose in the saliva (chew well!), as well as with pancreatic secretions. The resulting products (primarily disaccharide and oligosaccharide) are then broken down by enzymes (maltase) into glucose, a sugar used by the body to make energy. This takes place in the upper part of the small intestine cells; next, these sugars are channeled into mucous membrane cells. In stark contrast, when saccharose (as in table sugar or soft drinks, and so on.) is ingested, it is split into glucose and fructose (monosaccharides), which are immediately absorbed by the mucous membrane cell without any intestinal processing. Finally, there is milk sugar (lactose), which is processed by its own specific enzyme (lactase) in and around the intestinal cell. Milk sugar is metabolized much more slowly than the first two kinds of sugar.

So what does all this mean?

It means that eating different sources of sugar will result in very different levels of sugar in the blood—at completely different times. The speed at which carbohydrates are delivered into the small intestines for absorption is very important to your health.

This rate is regulated by the stomach, which can deliver its contents into the intestines either more or less rapidly. Mainly this is controlled by the kind of food that is consumed, although stress, irritation, composure, and relaxation also play a significant role. The larger the meal and the higher its fat content, the slower the stomach is emptied. Proteins reduce the stomach emptying time just a little, and carbohydrates, even less. Sweets and sugary drinks however pass through the stomach like a rocket, are quickly absorbed, and are transported to the liver in high concentration.

Remember our evolutionary tale: The liver wants to store glucose (as glycogen) for energy at a time of reduced food intake. But its capacity is limited; so whenever the intestine is flooded with glucose, an "unnatural" excess of glucose finds its way into the circulatory system.

This high blood sugar level triggers a strong release of insulin, leading to a rapid elimination of the glucose from the blood. The result?—At least 75 percent of the circulating glucose particles find their way to other tissues—particularly fat cells, which insulin then stimulates to build new fat. As if that wasn't enough, the rapid elimination of glucose from the blood leads to an earlier sense of fresh hunger.

And even that's not all: After the glucose reservoirs are full, all the consumed carbohydrates, which are no longer needed for energy, are also collected to build new fat (the liver can store only up to 50 or 100 grams of glycogen, muscle tissue only up to 200 or 300 grams). This new collection occurs partly in the liver, which forms new fat that is transported to fatty tissue as low-density serum cholesterol (VLDL), and stored. The remaining fat serves as the first stage of new LDL formation. And if excess free radicals enter the picture, or the inherited resistance against these aggressors is lacking, the deposits are increasingly oxidized. At this point we are taking giant steps towards developing the metabolic syndrome.

Let's summarize:

- All excess carbohydrate is used to form new fat.
- Rapidly absorbed sugars such as sucrose can form new

fat even before the glycogen reservoirs in the liver are filled. (This effect is slight when sucrose is used to sweeten food, but is very pronounced when sucrose is isolated or taken in connection with other carbohydrates, such as in the form of candy or sweet drinks.)

In practice, this means that for someone with an average energy requirement of 2,400 calories a day, 10 to 15 percent of the food consumed should be protein, 30 percent fat, and (only) 55 percent carbohydrates. Eat otherwise, and your diet can be dangerous.

One vitally important fact cannot be repeated enough—indeed it must be practically force-fed into modern man—humans cannot escape their genetic programming! Lucy's muscles were developed to make it possible for her to walk miles every day, in order to gather sufficient foodstuff, for herself and her baby, and to be able to fight or flee in the face of danger. Over the course of evolution, the body's need for this kind of behavior has been unshakably and undeniably genetically stamped into every single human being.

Up until about a hundred years ago, no problem. Most of the people in the West lived accordingly by doing hard physical labor earning a living in the fields, the forests, and later the factories. Their glucose reservoirs were periodically emptied and refilled. Aside from times of unusual food scarcity, or when only very limited nourishment was available, their food consumption remained generally in balance with their energy needs, sometimes slightly beneath it—the ideal situation according to nutritional scientists. (It has been known a long time, for example, that given two rat populations, one which is fattened, and one left hungry at times, the latter will be healthier by far and will live almost twice as long.)

Another important factor is that when there is an increased release of insulin, the normal regulated feelings of hunger and satiation controlled by the interbrain become disturbed. A downward spiral ensues that can lead to obesity at a breakneck speed: A constant excess of carbohydrates and high peaks in the blood sugar level trigger large insulin releases, which fills up the fatty tissue. Moreover, the constantly high insulin level causes a keen appetite. More and more is eaten, and each meal creates a deeper downward spiral anew. Since the controlling mechanism in the interbrain (adipostat) is constantly stimulated, stronger and stronger hunger attacks eventually lead to gorging. The whole system spirals gradually out of control and moves unavoidably to the final stage of metabolic syndrome.

The only way out of this crisis is to wind down the metabolism; this requires healthy weight reduction and a mild, gentle reprogramming of the adipostat—all the while avoiding the physiological state that will cause the notorious yo-yo effect. All of this will be achieved on the Turbo-Protein Diet.

WHAT'S THE ROLE
OF FREE RADICALS?

In order to correctly practice the protein diet, it's important to understand another phenomenon that increasingly threatens humans today. We are talking about free radicals. They represent the second largest threat to people enjoying a long, healthy life. Between the clashing rocks of Scylla (metabolic syndrome) and Charybdis (free radicals) lies the royal pathway to earthly paradise. A path that can only be trodden by the slim.

Free radicals are the aggressive interim products of our metabolism. They arise when a small portion of electrons do not form bonds during oxidation, but rather aimlessly wander around our bodies in search of something to react with. The body has its own defense system, the so-called "antioxidants," which attempt to eliminate these "metabolic terrorists." Some people seem to have a born resistance to free radicals. A particular gene or hormone (melatonin?) supposedly effects this resistance, which may guarantee longevity.

Free radicals are created during the oxygen exchange of normal breathing. These highly reactive particles are like a militant force with the worst designs on the commonwealth of the healthy body. Since they are extremely unstable they can trigger devastating chain reactions, and they are able to bond with many substances and structures in the human body.

If free radicals appear in excess amounts, they launch their first attack upon the cell surfaces, the membranes. The "antigen-determination" of every living being is located there. This simply means that the surface of every person's cells possesses a special, unique, personal code that can recognize the difference between its own (endogenic) and foreign (exogenic) substances, thus creating the basis for our immune defense system. As a result, our body can recognize every foreign protein that gets inside our body: bacteria, viruses, pollen, for example. When the body recognizes these outsiders, the enemy is attacked and destroyed so that the body can survive and remain healthy.

A conviction has grown that these particles are substantially involved in the hitherto unexplainable outbreak of certain diseases. Pancreatic cancer, for instance, is called free radical disease and can be successfully treated with antioxidants. No matter what form it may take, a constant bombarding of free radicals will cause some kind of serious disturbance in the equilibrium of the body, bringing illness in its wake.

When free radicals crack the code and penetrate the cell membrane, the tissue in question may suddenly perceive its own cells as intruders—and attacks them bitterly. The result is usually an autoimmune disease, where the body destroys its own tissue and there is no prospect of healing. In addition to allergies, such diseases include:

- crippling arthritis: The body attacks its own spinal chord and doesn't subsist until it is fully stiff and can no longer fulfill its functions.
- chronic polyarthritis: The body considers its own synovial (joint) membranes as a foreign substance and

rejects them, causing great pain.

- Colitis ulcerosa: The tissue of the large and small intestines is rejected creating painfully bleeding ulcers. Since the absorption of nutrition is no longer ensured, life is at risk.
- many nerve diseases as well (multiple sclerosis for example).

These disorders should be fully considered under a new light with free radicals in mind.

Once the free radicals have paved a destructive path deeper into the cell, they come up against the organelles and burst their membranes. This is an assault on the hereditary substance within the cell nucleus and leads to changes in the nucleic acid (DNS). As mentioned elsewhere, after an excessive consumption of high-calorie food (too much fat, too many carbohydrates) LDL and VLDL cholesterol are increasingly oxidized by an excess of free radicals. The results include cardiovascular diseases, reduced quality of life, and a shortened life expectancy.

In order to inactivate the free radicals, the body is equipped with antioxidants as part of its defense system. One must distinguish two types:

- Enzymatic antioxidants that require trace elements such as zinc, copper, manganese, and selenium in order to function, and
- Non-enzymatic antioxidants that serve as hydrogen donors and render the free radicals harmless by neutralization. The most important of these are vitamin C, vitamin E, and beta-carotene (provitamin A).

Food rich in vitamins, trace elements, and minerals provides the best protection against attacks from free radicals. Furthermore, stimulating the metabolism favors both the production and the effectiveness of antioxidants. First and foremost, however: Don't eat too much, since the more food is consumed, the more oxidants (free radicals) are set free.

The consumption of both nicotine and alcohol have an extremely negative influence on the supply of antioxidants. On the one hand smokers and heavy drinkers need more antioxidants than those who abstain, on the other hand they usually live on a diet considerably less rich in vitamins and minerals. Also, extensive sunbathing, high ozone levels, airplane trips, chemotherapy, contact with heavy metals (lead, cadmium, mercury), and eating food grown in overfertilized soils (selenium deficiency) can also contribute to an excess of free radicals.

If one doesn't belong to a particularly endangered group of regular nicotine and alcohol consumers, one can assume that the body gets sufficient antioxidants if it is fed about a pound of vegetables every day. Vegetable juices are a good alternative for those who don't like to cook. Vitamin tablets should be taken as a last resort. Make sure your diet contains plenty of the necessary vitamins and minerals, so that the free radicals don't have a chance to attack your health. It is often very difficult to repair serious damage to healthy cells once this has already occurred.

It has been proven that the following vitamins and trace elements are effective killers of free radicals:

- Beta-carotene (provitamin A): Contained in yellow and green vegetables and fruits, it is extremely heat and light sensitive. The ideal preparation is a salad dressed with a bit of oil, so that fat-soluble carotene can be more effectively taken up by the body.

- Vitamin A: Found in milk products, eggs, liver, and fish, it is also heat sensitive.
- Vitamin C: It is contained in citrus fruits and sweet peppers. It is destroyed by long storage times and over cooking.
- Vitamin E: Good sources are wheat germ oil and sun flower seeds, as well as beef and pork. This vitamin is heat resistant and can survive most moderate cooking methods without damage.
- Zinc, copper, selenium: These trace elements help the body's own antioxidants protect healthy cells. They are found in shellfish, poultry, and especially in innards (for instance liver). Ocean fish are rich in selenium.
- Garlic, leeks, onions, and all vegetables of the cabbage family (for instance broccoli) contain antioxidants that remain intact after moderate cooking.

It is important to limit possible free radical damage with antioxidants when attempting to lose excess weight by dieting. As we shall soon see (see page 56), too many free radicals in the blood can greatly hinder the conversion of the thyroid hormone T_4 into the active T_3, causing the whole metabolic process to slow down. A sluggish metabolism causes increasingly more fat to be put on.

When in doubt, using a blood test to determine the quantity of free radicals in an individual is recommended, and medical treatment should be initiated if necessary. But refrain from every uncontrolled self-medication with vitamin and mineral preparations!

NO PAIN, NO GAIN

The goal of this book is to explain a diet, which will allow you to lose weight sensibly and healthily under the given physiological conditions, to put a stop to the yo-yo effect, and even train your body to maintain a stable weight.

From a point of view of biological medicine (practiced more in Europe, similar to what's often called holistic medicine in the U.S.), it is impossible to lose weight in a healthy manner using limited caloric intake as the only means. Achieving a healthy, lasting weight loss is a complex process that will do your body a real service, helping it in many other ways. Our evolution has placed humans in a relatively tight corset of physiological givens that cannot simply be cast off without doing serious damage.

Let's think back to our ancient foremother Lucy, and her clan, and consider the biological conditions and proscriptions in which she lived.

As already described, Lucy was forced to constantly search for food in order to survive. Confronted with danger, she had to either flee quickly or fight for her life. Let's be perfectly clear—this reaction pattern and the attendant physiological processes still apply to us today—on another plane and in different contexts to be sure, but these reactions occur all the time to ensure that humans remain healthy and survive.

Keeping this in mind, let's take a look at our muscular apparatus. What is its biological purpose? First of all, it makes movement possible—the decisive prerequisite for the search of food. Mankind would have long since become extinct, if its individuals couldn't cover long stretches of ground in the search of appropriate food. And without a sophisticated mobility, flight in times of danger would have been impossible as well. Muscles also provide the ability to fight, another survival strategy at man's disposal since earliest times. The evolutionary purpose is clear: muscle movement preserves the species.

The energy needed for these sweaty tasks and harrowing adventures is provided to the muscles by the stored glucose. To understand how this works, it is important to know that innumerable receptors (receivers) on the inner and outer surface of every muscle cell control glucose transport into the cell to create energy. In order to function properly, this transport must be ongoing and vigorous, which is exactly what happened for millions of years during the natural survival process. People didn't know of any way to live except by hard physical exertion. By physical work they made their livelihood and cared for their offspring. And it all served to further evolution.

Up until about a hundred years ago, most people had these glucose receptors so fully trained that cardiovascular and metabolic diseases were practically unknown. But the industrial revolution, sweeping technological developments, and now the electronic revolution have fundamentally transformed the daily life of modern man. One gets the impression that our muscles are only exerted in fitness studios nowadays—for some people, muscles are used only for picking up a pack of cigarettes or opening a can of beer. No one seems alarmed that almost every man over 40 and every second woman over 55 suffers from some form of a civilization sickness. This term even plays down the dangers of such diseases, which for instance cost the German economy alone the equivalent of 80 billion dollars annually. And the tendency for these illnesses is rising.

Sure, the beer and a steak taste mighty good, and for some, possibly the cigarette afterwards while comfortably watching TV, but life expectancy and increasingly quality of life as well are clearly restricted by civilization illnesses. Moreover, the conviction that we can "trick" our biological destiny with the help of chemistry and pharmaceuticals is deceptive. Only one thing really helps—common sense eating and a radical about-face towards more exercise.

THE METABOLIC SYNDROME

I n order to better understand the complex processes involved, we will examine the metabolic syndrome in greater detail.

The metabolic syndrome has four aspects:
- A high blood sugar level with increased insulin production,
- High blood pressure,
- Arteriosclerosis and fat metabolism disturbances, and
- Diabetes mellitus.

We already know that when Lucy is under stress, fleeing or fighting, glucose must be pumped into her muscle cells to provide necessary energy, once the available carbohydrates have been all used up. We know that this takes place by means of certain receptors. The mechanism of these receptors is so vitally important to our survival that it must be constantly stimulated or its action will be stunted. Since we possess a great variety and diversity of muscles, considerable effort is necessary to sufficiently activate all receptors. This occurs with hard physical labor or intensive sports activity.

If this kind activity is absent, a "down regulation" of the receptors comes to pass; in other words, they become reduced in number and lose their effectiveness. The receptors become increasingly less sensitive, until finally no glucose can be released to the muscles at all. As a result, the blood sugar level rises. The pancreas then releases more insulin.

A high level of insulin is fatal in two ways. On one hand, the body interprets the situation as lack of nourishment, and therefore releases more fat from its storage deposits. The drastically rising levels of cholesterol and triglyceride in the blood eventually lead to blood vessel deposits, and thus to vascular restriction. The threat of a heart attack or stroke is the result. On the other hand, insulin acts as a growth stimulant on the arterial walls and heart.

The blood vessels are hence doubly under stress. As deposits and restriction (arteriosclerosis) increase, blood pressure rises, and the heart size enlarges. This leads to heart weakness once the critical heart weight has reached or surpassed 500 grams. The pumping power of the heart is restricted, bodily performance drops, and the quality of life is drastically reduced. Medication can only insufficiently compensate for all this.

If no efficient countermeasures such as diet and increased exercise are taken, the negative downward spiral gets worse and worse: Higher insulin levels stimulate strong hunger pangs; the ignorant and suffering human eats more and more. The pancreas is exhausted and gets behind on its insulin production. And the dead end is soon reached: diabetes mellitus.

All four components of metabolic syndrome—high blood sugar level along with increased insulin production, high blood pressure, arteriosclerosis and fat metabolism disturbances, and diabetes mellitus—lead to a drastic reduction in life expectancy and quality of life. These conditions are insidiously dangerous, because for a long time nothing really hurts, so no mental trauma instigates taking action against them. We will escape from this metabolic inferno only when we consider fundamental survival principles and lead a more active life. Since hard physical labor is no longer a part of the ordinary work day for most of us, the only sensible alternative is some sport that we can actively enjoy.

It should be clear that exercise is only really valuable when it produces beads of sweat! The glucose stored in the muscles must be effectively emptied; the glucose receptor power plants demand intensive training. Accordingly it is currently believed that only sports can produce the necessary physiological effect of demanding at least 80 percent of one's maximum output. The motto applies: No pain, no gain.

American scientists carried out a comprehensive 20-year study on 17,300 healthy people; it demonstrated that adding an active sport to your lifestyle was rewarded with a 26 percent reduction in the death rate. From this example, one may surmise that those who burn up at least 1,500 calories a week in energetic training will benefit from it. Exercise alone will do the job; it can heat up the metabolic rate six times above normal. Moderate jogging can burn up around 600 to 700 calories, and an increased pace can easily double that per hour.

The controversial question whether intensive sports activity increases life expectancy is to be answered with a definite yes—assuming that a minimal weekly performance fulfills certain requirements (for instance, jogging 20 miles, or playing tennis for three hours). The most sensible course is to combine very dynamic sports such as jogging, bicycling, or swimming- with floor exercises.

Life should be enjoyable, so don't go to the other extreme either and plague yourself with a regimen of constant exercise. After all, we're talking about enhanced quality of life here, which is more valuable than all the good advice in the world, and so must never be ignored. One doesn't have to train the body every day. In fact it is the contrast between effort and relaxation that is so appealing, which corresponds more to our own natural biological rhythms, and thus is physiologically a more sensible approach.

Looking after one's psyche is another especially important component of good health that cannot be overlooked. When sport is intense enough to bring up a sweat, a certain "high" results from the release of endorphins (internal morphine), often triggering euphoria or even ecstasy. The pain threshold is raised as well. One can become hooked on this homemade good mood: As soon as the hormone level sinks in the blood, one longs to exercise again. This is probably the least dangerous form of dependency on earth.

Anyone who trains his or her body in such a way will very quickly enjoy a completely new physical awareness, instinctively taking a healthier diet, avoiding unhealthy habits, and becoming less susceptible to all kinds of sickness as a result. An ounce of prevention is worth a pound of cure. Even when the first symptoms of metabolic syndrome appear, the sensitivity of the receptors can be restimulated by physical activity. Don't overdo it in the beginning; start out with a gradually increasing training program (beginning on page 85).

Intensive exercise is a fundamental prerequisite for health and longevity. Another important factor is maintaining your normal weight, which will be reestablished and preserved with this diet. Being overweight is generally the result of both overeating and too little exercise or energy consumption. The oft-cited "glands" are very rarely—only in a few exceptional cases—the cause of obesity. Yet it is a good idea to take a closer look at the metabolic processes that play an important role in gaining and losing weight, especially those controlled by the thyroid gland.

WHAT YOU MUST KNOW
ABOUT YOUR METABOLISM

The thyroid gland is the central organ of our metabolism. Any serious weight-reduction diet must be based on a knowledge of its function.

The thyroid gland consists of two flaps located on the left and right of the larynx. As with almost all hormone systems, it is embedded within a feedback mechanism. The cerebrum gives commands to release thyroid hormones, which then have an effect on specific target organs. Two varieties of thyroid hormones are released: T_4 and T_3.

T_4 (tetra-iodothyronine, or thyroxin) can be considered a preliminary stage of the active metabolic hormone T_3 (tri-iodothyronine). T_4 competes with the nearly identical (except for one iodine atom) T_3 to reach the receptors that lie primarily in the skin, muscles, and fatty tissue—where the central metabolic processes take place after T_4 has been converted to T_3 by the enzyme de-iodase. The basal metabolism (the level of energy consumption at rest) rises, fat is burned, and more warmth is produced.

Our body produces relatively more T_4 than T_3 hormone. This applies a brake on the rate of metabolic processes because T_3 is five times stronger. Thus our bodies are protected from consuming energy too quickly, and we can build up a padding of fat as reserve for bad times. During this process, as we will see in detail later, the adipostat in the interbrain functions as an important controller. Thanks to this biological equipment, mankind has survived for millions of years despite extreme famines and crises.

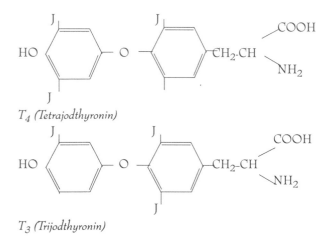

T_4 (Tetrajodthyronin)

T_3 (Trijodthyronin)

Certain foods can influence the conversion of T_4 into T_3, particularly protein, which causes increased amounts of the enzyme de-iodase to be produced, followed by increased transformation of T_4 into T_3. But this conversion is limited by the average protein content of our primary protein sources. For instance, in 100 grams of curd, there are only 15 to 20 grams of protein. In order to convert greater amounts of T_4 into T_3 due to protein intake, enormous quantities of food would have to be consumed, which would also contain an unhealthy amount of animal fat. The limited space and digestive capacity of our stomach and intestinal tract makes this impossible however. Nevertheless our special diet program can take advantage of this effect!

It is important to emphasize that for us, protein is the most valuable building block. It cannot be replaced. When we consume protein-rich food, our bodies are in the position to burn more calories with increased efficiency. If our diet contains less protein and times are not so rosy, our bodily organism turns down its metabolic pump and saves energy for the future. This is how evolution has kept *Homo sapiens* from extinction to this day.

Basal Metabolism and Protein

Basal metabolism is the energy consumption of a sober person over a 24-hour period while resting in a prone position. The basal metabolism of an average adult is calculated as follows:

- 1 pound of body weight resting for 1 hour uses ½ calorie,
- 1 pound of body weight resting for 24 hours uses 11 calories,
- So, for example, a 150-pound person resting for 24 hours would use 1650 calories.

Basal metabolism depends not so much on the absolute body weight, but rather on the relationship between body weight and body surface. A mouse, for instance, has a relatively high metabolism compared to a human, since it has more surface area per pound. The greater the surface area compared to the weight, the higher the metabolism. In other words, the more heat given off, the more heat needed in order to maintain body temperature.

Aside from the body's surface area, the basal metabolism is primarily influenced by the thyroid gland. Thyroid hyperactivity (over functioning) raises the basal metabolism, and hypoactivity (retarded functioning) lowers it. Age and sex also help determine the basal metabolism, which sinks with increased age. Women have a 10 percent lower basal metabolism than men.

Even the slightest muscle movement—even a fever—can increase basal metabolism. A little muscle movement daily increases metabolism by 550 calories, moderate work about 1,130 calories. Eating causes an increase both in oxygen intake and carbon dioxide output, but this occurs to a much smaller degree than with muscle power. But the decisive factor is the kind of nourishment consumed. Protein stimulates basal metabolism the best: 20 to 30 percent; carbohydrates are less effective: 5 to 8 percent; followed by fats: 2 to 4 percent. The effect of nutritional substances on basal metabolism, called the "specific–dynamic effect," is always most powerful when the diet is rich in valuable essential amino acids (protein) that the body needs daily and cannot produce itself—and without which no higher biological function is imaginable.

These protein building blocks are of decisive importance for:
- The thyroid and sex hormones,
- The neurotransmitters that control the switching processes between nerves and muscles and that can produce either a pleasurable feeling of contentment, or depression, and
- The enzymes, which catalyze and therefore control the entire metabolism.

Furthermore, numerous other important body systems depend on the influx of protein substances. Aside from the eight essential amino acids, the body must be supplied with a number of other protein components that also stimulate the metabolism. The specific–dynamic effect can generally be maintained for up to six hours. Perhaps you have noticed that on hot days you sweat longer than usual after consuming a protein-rich meal.

Remember: Without the interaction between our organism and essential amino acids there would be no highly differentiated life forms, no activity or reproduction would be possible, and no organism could remain healthy in the long run. This applies to any weight-reducing diet, no matter what kind. It's not surprising that every year countless people damage their bodies, even die, from the effects of erroneously conceived diets that do not take fundamental physiological laws into account.

No matter what, a healthy body cannot survive without at least ½ gram of protein daily for every pound of body weight, with moderate exercise. An ideal meal contains approximately:

- 12 to 15 percent protein,
- 30 percent fat, and
- 55 percent carbohydrate.

This combination results in a relatively slow emptying of the stomach. The insulin level, which to a large degree determines the sensation of hunger, only rises gradually. As a result, a fairly long phase of satiation is attained, while the body obtains its proper daily ration of about 2,400 calories, which certainly does not contribute to fat deposits in the average person.

If this rule of thumb is not observed, and a greater percentage of carbohydrates is consumed, there is a danger of creating fat deposits. If furthermore the body receives a constant influx of sweet snacks such as chocolate bars and soft drinks, the blood sugar level rises dramatically. When these levels sink abruptly, the person is plagued by keen pangs of hunger, which leads to more eating, even though the day's total ration of calories has been consumed long ago.

DIET, STRESS AND THE YO-YO EFFECT

B y now it should be clear that the human body, following an evolutionary survival strategy that has successfully maintained the species up until now, only taps its fat reserves in an extreme emergency. This won't happen if you do nothing except reduce your calorie intake. On the contrary, your body will set off all its alarm bells in such a case: "Warning, warning! Mortal danger due to starvation!"

This alarm triggers stress of the worst kind, since the body's primary concern is survival. Feverishly a flood of stress hormones is released, cortisol being the most important. The main effect of cortisol is its influence on the carbohydrate, protein, and to a less extent fat metabolism.

Unfortunately, the released cortisol makes glucose available from the protein storage depots in the muscles and heart, not from the fat deposits. Free fatty acids are partially mobilized for energy, but the main action is from proteins. The muscle mass is melted down, and fats circulate in the blood— only to be deposited again as soon as the hunger period (diet) is over. The redepositing of fat often occurs in different areas of the body than before the diet, an effect that particularly plagues women—causing the shape that makes pants ride up for instance.

The Result: After a conventional weight-reducing diet, we have less muscle, generally feel worse, and the ugly fat cushions are still there, possibly in worse places! The body's reaction to food deprivation and hunger is automatic. Experts call this process "aminoplastic gluconeogenesis," although the ordinary person eager to lose weight usually just calls it frustrating.

And the next grievous problem already looms on the horizon: The glucose obtained from metabolizing muscle tissue inevitably raises the insulin level in the blood. Once again the high insulin level creates hunger pangs! Stress is increased and becomes continuous since the dieter must now exercise great self-discipline day and night to resist the attacks of hunger.

Now the body's protein environment is entirely out of balance. Emaciated bones become brittle, the skin loses its texture, and the muscles their elasticity. Cortisol can also damage connective tissue and impede its regeneration. Women are especially susceptible to the negative side effects of conventional weight loss diets; often their skin becomes wrinkled and marked with unattractive stripes. Another unfortunate side effect of conventional diets is the increased susceptibility to infections.

Since cortisol also tends to raise blood pressure, every overweight person should consult a doctor before beginning a diet. In fact, the optimal solution would be careful supervision on the part of the physician during the entire diet, in order to avoid damaging side effects. A diet should never result in reduced weight at the cost of good health.

Since the body automatically assumes that there is a threat of starvation during reduced caloric intake, it will slow metabolism as much as it can. So, at the same time the dieter is enduring stressful species-preserving hunger attacks, the thyroid gland, which is the central metabolic controlling device, receives the command to massively save energy reserves. Similar to hibernation, the thyroid drastically throttles all the metabolic processes, attempting to give the body a better chance of surviving food deprivation.

Initially, a person on a diet generally experiences success, but in truth, it is only muscle mass and water that is lost. Afterwards hardly another pound goes away, or a certain weight plateau is reached. Further suffering with continued fasting only stimulates the down regulation of the metabolism even more. Then there is even less weight loss, but stress and hunger increase incessantly.

If the fast is broken and normal food is consumed again, the rate of weight gain is now doubled due to the reduced metabolic rate. Often, the poor victim plunges into another fad diet, setting the disastrous spiral into motion once again. The heart and circulatory system, as well as the immune system, suffer the most as a result. In the end this yo-yo effect is a mortally dangerous matter. Since the Turbo-Protein Diet is designed to make use of the normal metabolic processes, it avoids the dreaded yo-yo effect, which dooms conventional diets to failure.

THE REGULATION OF FAT GAIN: OB-GENE AND ADIPOSTAT

The extent of fat gain is largely prescribed by the controlling center in the interbrain, the adipostat, where the body's target fat level is stored. The adipostat's task is to continuously compare the target value with the actual amount in the body, and if necessary bring them into accord. If the person is deprived of food—whether because of famine or a conscious weight-reduction diet—the hormone leptin sets off the alarm in the adipostat.

According to the latest research, we know that chromosome number seven carries the information that governs an individual's fat distribution. There is a special inherited characteristic found there called the "ob-gene" (obesity gene), which controls feelings of hunger and satiation. This gene stimulates the fat cells to produce the leptin (from leptos: thin, slender). The more fat there is, the more leptin is synthesized. When the leptin level is high, the enzyme de-iodase (mentioned in connection with the thyroid gland) is also produced in greater quantities. The thyroid gland, after all, is also a part of this complicated, ingenious feedback mechanism. The body then feels less hungry, so that less food is consumed. At the same time, increased bodily activity is stimulated by the sympathetic nervous system.

Fat Regulation

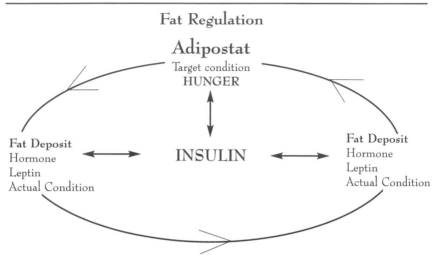

Auto regulation of fat storage in humans.

But what a disaster if the leptin level sinks because of a diet! Low leptin plus the constantly high insulin level signals the adipostat to reestablish an appropriate balance. So it does—by triggering sharp hunger cravings and eating frenzies; the adipostat demands that the fat depots are refilled in the shortest possible time. Only then will it leave the body in peace. During this race to catch up on fat storage, less de-iodase is produced by the thyroid gland, and this stress situation can trigger the aforementioned massive release of cortisol. Only a very small percentage of overweight and obese people have a defective ob-gene. These people suffer from thick pads of fat from early childhood; their high insulin levels create a constant feeling of hunger. Satiation is never attained, since the controlling mechanisms never come into harmony with the body.

The common vernacular glosses over the true clinical picture by talking about a "glandular dysfunction," or medical experts talk about "adiposity." People diagnosed with genuine adiposity need long-term care, and they suffer early from metabolic syndrome. But the overwhelming majority of overweight people have simply accumulated too much fat by eating too much rich food, and they are in the position to get rid of these excess pounds on their own. The Turbo-Protein Diet effectively supports those who are willing to do so in a sensible and healthy manner. The secret of the diet's success is that it takes all the body's natural physiological processes into account, and puts them into service for losing excess weight.

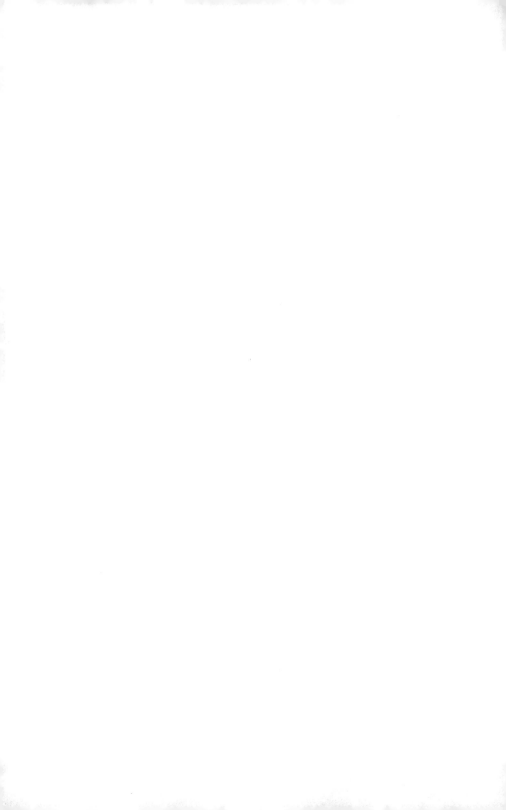

Part Two

Healthy Weight Reduction:
The Turbo-Protein Diet

What You Must Know Beforehand

The Turbo-Protein Diet is a pure liquid fast cure that can be carried out at home. It is supplemented with a simple exercise program.

Healthy adults under 35 years of age, who are no more than 45 pounds overweight, but who are used to at least a minimum of athletic training, can begin this diet at once.

People more than 45 pounds overweight, and those who are sick, "couch potatoes," adolescents, or women who are pregnant, should first go to their physician and undergo a thorough check-up before starting the diet and an accompanying sports program. People with cardiovascular, circulatory, or thyroid problems as well as diabetics, or those who must regularly take medication, should as a matter of course participate in a diet program only under a physician's watchful care.

Eager beavers can aim for a target weight in the lower range of the Body Mass Index (see page 32). But one should always keep in mind that the ideal weight is what feels good—the weight where you have peak performance and where you feel you are in good shape.

SLENDER AND FIT
WITH LIQUID NOURISHMENT

You do not consume any solid food on the Turbo-Protein Diet. Your nourishment consists entirely of a drink made of special soy milk protein and a honey enzyme, and vegetable broth.

The powder preparation used in the diet drink is about two thirds vegetable protein, and one third animal protein. It has been pre-fermented by a honey enzyme supplement and can thus be easily absorbed by the body. The 53 percent protein content is considerably higher than conventional supplements, which generally offer only 15 to 20 percent protein. This protein drink supplies the body with a large dose of easily digestible pure protein, in a form not normally available in food. Remember: while losing weight, the body must be provided with the essential amino acids, otherwise serious health problems can occur!

The vegetable broth gives you sufficient antioxidants to neutralize any free radicals, which is sensible nutrition all by itself, but is extremely useful in conjunction with an accompanying sports program. Poorly balanced meals do not generally provide most people with enough antioxidants. Exercise, on the other hand, favors free radical formation because the body metabolizes about twenty times more oxygen under strain, than it does at rest.

Both the protein drink and vegetable broth cause rapid weight loss simply by attacking fat deposits. This creates an "anti-yo-yo effect."

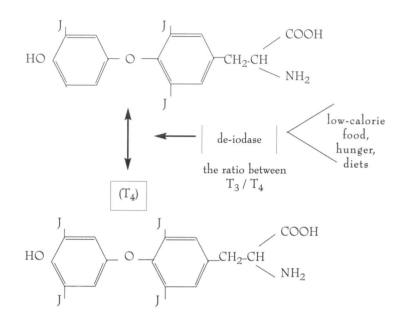

Yo-Yo Effect: This is the alarm reaction to hunger and fasting, and is a typical response to most weight-loss regimens.

The yo-yo effect is characterized by:
- Reduced synthesis of T_4
- A decline in de-iodase activity
- Down regulation (restraining) of the metabolic rate
  —in order to gain valuable "survival time."

Liquid protein's unique composition causes:
- A relaxation of the gastrointestinal tract, and
- A switching off of the adipostat, which prevents the release of cortisol with all its negative consequences, including the attack on the body's vital protein reserves in the muscle and heart.

The *Anti*-Yo-Yo Effect is characterized by:
- The high specific–dynamic effect of protein,
- Increased formation of T_4,
- A high conversion rate of T_4 into T_3,

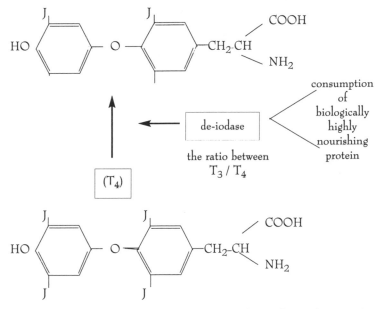

The Anti-Yo-Yo Effect: high specific–dynamic effect of protein ➤ *increased formation of T_4 and high conversion rates of T_4 and T_3* ➤ *stimulation of the metabolism* ➤ *significant weight lost*

- Significant weight loss from fat burning,
- A lower insulin level so hunger pangs are severely reduced, and
- A stimulation of the thyroid gland that switches off the metabolic conditions that create the yo-yo effect.

The constant supply of highly concentrated protein mixture that can be absorbed extremely easily by the body prevents the "Warning! Danger due to food deficiency! alarm" from going off. Instead of melting off the usual protein reserves (muscles, heart) in order to obtain quick energy in the form of sugar (glucose), the body now burns the proper safety reserves for energy—fat. This process is enhanced by plenty of exercise.

WARNING: Any solid food consumed during a liquid fast cure—even yogurt or a small apple—will inevitably cause the production of digestive juices and therefore insulin, thereby stimulating the adipostat. Consequently, all the desired mechanisms for specific fat reduction will fail. So remain steadfast, and follow the diet exactly as directed!

THE FIRST DAY
OF THE FAST

Before starting the fast, you must purchase one or two cans of the special protein mixture, Almased-Vitalkost. This is the enzyme product that has proven so effective with my patients. Fortunately "Almased," as it is called, is available in the U.S., possibly at health food stores, but definitely at the address listed at the end of this book. Also stock up with a healthy supply fresh vegetables for the broth, particularly those rich in vitamins E and C and beta carotene, such as tomatoes, carrots, broccoli, leeks, onions, potatoes, and peppers. If you don't have time to cook, you can rely on instant vegetable broth.

Begin your diet on a free, quiet day with nothing particular on your schedule.

It's absolutely necessary that a toilet be nearby, since the first step in reducing weight is a thorough evacuation of the bowels.

Prepare a laxative. (Any fast-acting over-the-counter laxative is suitable.) Or, an enema will have the same effect.

About two hours later you will feel the effect, and depending on how full your intestinal tract was, you will have several bowel movements (up to five or so). Afterwards you may feel a light stomach colic, and perhaps your mood will sink to an absolute zero. But all that passes quickly. Keep your goal in mind and don't give up! If necessary, repeat this procedure every 3 to 4 days. Start taking the protein drink on this same day. Usual medication can be continued.

THE PROTEIN DRINK

Take the Almased three times a day. It is simple to take the correct amount. One slightly heaping teaspoon corresponds to 2.5 grams of protein. You should take about one-half gram of protein per pound of "normal" body weight (your target body weight, not your current body weight!). The calculation is simple, simply take your target body weight in pounds, and divide this by 5 to get the daily requirement. For example: A person weighing 150 pounds would figure 150 lbs ÷ 5 = 30 slightly heaping teaspoons of protein powder daily.

Divide the calculated daily requirement of protein powder into three portions, so you can take one third of the total in the morning, one third at noon, and one third at night. Mix the powder with water to make a drink. For example: Our 150-pound person would divide the daily ration of 30 teaspoons of protein powder into three portions of 10 teaspoons each: to drink in the morning, at noon, and in the evening.

If you so desire, you can mix the slightly nutty-tasting protein drink with some tea, coffee, low-fat milk, or (sugar-free!) flavored water instead of bottled or tap water. Just remember—every additional calorie consumed slows down the weight-reducing process. Forty grams of protein powder equals 130 calories. Almased can lower your blood sugar level (and cholesterol).

THE VEGETABLE COCKTAIL

I deally, one should prepare a fresh vegetable broth every day. Simply cut about half a pound of the vitamin-rich vegetables such as carrots, peppers, tomatoes, broccoli, leeks, onions, or potatoes into cubes, then add 1.5 to 2 quarts of water and cook for about five minutes in a pressure cooker, or longer in a normal pot, until soft. Pour the finished vegetable broth through a strainer, filter out the solid pieces, which can be frozen and eaten at a later date.

IMPORTANT: Once again, this diet's success depends on you to NOT TAKE ANY SOLID FOOD during the duration of the diet. Do not yield to the temptation of eating the delicious solid vegetable pieces now! Medications you ordinarily take are continued as usual.

You may season the clear vegetable broth, but go very easy on the salt. It is best if you refrain from salt altogether, and season the broth only with appropriate herbs. You can sip this broth, or an instant vegetable broth, all day long. For added flavor, dissolve one effervescent multivitamin tablet in water and combine with one portion of Almased powder or supplement the program with a multi-vitamin.

Drink Sufficient Liquids

The vegetable broth is an important source of liquid. Nevertheless, you must consume a total daily amount of 3 to 3.5 quarts of fluid. So every day, drink as much uncarbonated water or unsweetened herb tea as you can. You are also allowed to drink coffee and black tea during the diet, although these drinks are not well suited for cleaning out your system and rapidly losing weight. Avoid alcoholic beverages, since they put too much of a strain on your metabolism and contain far too many calories.

IMPORTANT: Be sure to conscientiously control your liquid intake during the diet. You pay a high price for drinking too little while fasting—metabolic poisoning and kidney disease.

STIMULATE YOUR METABOLISM
WITH EXERCISE

While you are losing weight on the Turbo-Protein Diet, you will notice that your whole body switches over from the sympathetic nervous system, the "driver," to the parasympathetic nervous system, the "quieting nerves." Your heart beats more calmly, your pulse is slower, and your blood pressure decreases. In general you will feel somewhat less energetic and more sluggish. So, don't rush into anything hastily and remain calm.

In order to get your body going to accomplish the day's tasks, it's necessary to kick-start the circulation and muscles a little with exercise. This will regulate your blood pressure and provide a sense of well-being as well.

Endorphins are released while you exercise. Their effect is strengthened by ketone bodies produced during the massive fat combustion taking place during the diet cure. Just like the endorphins, they give you a sense of elation. Many patients have reported an incredible burst of energy even after the first protein drink, followed by an intense feeling of well-being, which is surely rooted in the very high nutritional value of the protein powder. Thus, you have now begun to take the advantage of the turbo effect of the Turbo-Protein Diet.

The sports program is divided into two sections: floor exercises, which build muscle and raise basal metabolism, and jogging, bicycle riding, or swimming, which improve stamina and performance capacity. The exercises should be done two to three times a week. Those who are already well trained are of course free to do the exercises daily from the start, and truly exert themselves.

The Floor Exercises

The recommended exercises primarily work the stomach and back muscles, as well as the arm and leg muscles.

- Try to find your own rhythm with these exercises and attempt to intensify your workout every day.
- How often you do the exercises depends on your physi cal condition. A general rule of thumb is to repeat every exercise as many times as you can, so long as you have control, even if the muscle begins to tremble or burn.
- And never forget to maintain regular breathing while you exercise: Do not hold your breath, even while under the greatest physical strain.

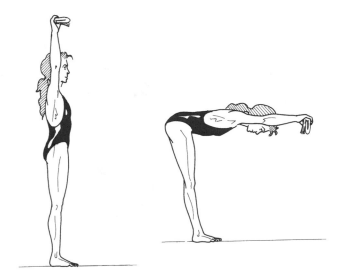

1. Exercising the stomach and back:

You need two equally heavy books or magazines for this exercise. Stand upright with legs slightly apart and the knees slightly bent. Hold a book or rolled up magazine in your hands. Bend forward to form a right angle with your body, stretching your arms out straight in front of you; then, straighten up slowly, with a powerfully controlled movement, until your arms point up to the ceiling. Then once again, slowly bend your upper torso forward. Repeat this exercise as many times as you can. Remember to breathe steadily. Avoid rocking back and forth with rapid, swinging movements—it is more effective to work your muscles slowly and powerfully.

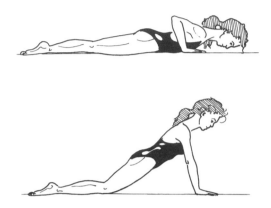

2. Exercising the arms, shoulders, chest, and back:

Lie down on your stomach, supporting yourself on your hands just below the shoulders. Tighten the stomach muscles and push yourself slowly upwards and back down again, without ever letting your body rest with its full weight on the floor.

Men do these push-ups with stretched legs, their weight on their toes. Women should let their calves rest on the ground, or they can also support themselves on their knees and cross their feet in the air. These push-ups are very strenuous, but extremely effective. For a start, force yourself to do at least three, and then try to increase this number as time goes by. Don't forget to breathe!

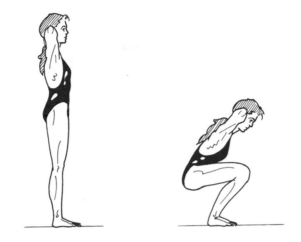

3. Exercising the thighs:

Stand with your legs spread wide apart and your knees slightly bent. Fold your hands behind your head. Lower yourself slowly into a crouch. The upper torso remains upright, the back straight. Look forward. Push your rear end back while going down, as if you wanted to sit on a chair. Then come slowly back up, but without totally straightening the knees. Repeat this exercise slowly and under great control, until your strength gives out. Take care that your leg muscles do the work; the upper torso remains still.

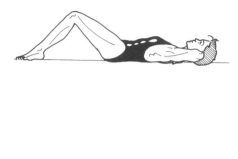

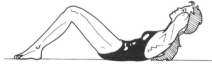

4. Exercise for the stomach:

Lie down on your back, placing your feet comfortably on the floor. Press your spine down to the floor, and fold your hands behind your head. Your elbows should point outward and not upwards, and your chin should face the ceiling. Lift and lower your head and shoulders with the help of your stomach muscles. Your head should not touch the floor when lowered, and your chin should always face the ceiling. Breathe out as you rise, breathe in as you come back down.

Do this exercise as long as you can, even if you feel your muscles burning. It is very important that your spinal cord touches the floor during the entire exercise.

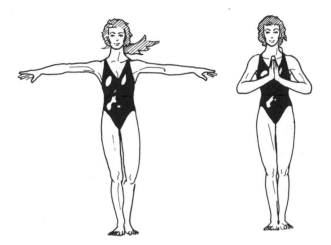

5. Final exercise:

Always finish your gymnastic training program by spinning rapidly around on your own axis like a dervish with outstretched arms. Watch out: Always turn only to the right! Stop spinning simply by slowing down your turns. When you come to a stop, pause and press the palms of your hands together at your breast, about at the height of your heart.

At first you might feel dizzy even after one or two spins. But don't get discouraged! Keep practicing until you have spun around on your own axis a few times without losing your balance, and you can finish the exercise in a controlled manner.

This particular exercise helps you to synchronize the right and left sides of your brain. Afterwards you will be more intuitive and creative, and your emotional world will be intensified.

Stamina training for the heart and circulatory system

Sports such as running, jogging, swimming, or bicycling are good for building stamina. Choose the kind of stamina training that appeals to you most, since enjoyment is the best assurance you will continue your program.

With jogging it's important not to overexert yourself, but to breathe well, and only slowly increase your stamina with longer runs. At first you might feel like you're not getting anywhere at all, or that you have to take a break after only a minute or two. Don't worry about it! Find your own rhythm and improve your performance gradually, step by step.

The most effective training takes place when you exert yourself until you reach about 80 percent of your maximum capability. It's to your advantage if you sweat profusely during your workouts.

During your diet cure, take the time to work out intensively in the sport of your choice at least three times a week. You lose weight a lot faster this way, and do your body a good service as well.

LENGTH OF THE DIET
AND THE SUCCESS RATE

I f you heed all the instructions for the Turbo-Protein Diet and conscientiously carry out the sports program, you will be rewarded with a true weight loss of one-half to one pound every day. Your fat padding will disappear, instead of just stored water or muscle tissue.

A loss of about 6 to 9 pounds a week is the rule. In two weeks you can lose 12 to 18 pounds, depending on your constitution. This equals a total of 50,000 calories.

I urge you—don't attempt a major weight loss too rapidly in one attempt; remember that your skin has to adjust to the new situation. If you try to go too fast, unsightly "stripes" appear in the soft connecting tissue, particularly for women. It is much better to take off 10 to 20 pounds; then take a break for a few weeks before starting the diet again. This is much healthier.

If the pounds don't fall off as fast as you would expect from reading all this information, it could be because thyroid hormone is not being converted from T_4 into T_3 due to excess free radicals. A physician's opinion should be relied upon to determine whether antioxidants should eventually be prescribed.

BREAKING THE FAST

After one to two weeks of the fasting cure as described, or when the first 10 to 20 pounds have been taken off, return to your normal eating habits. Don't do this suddenly, however! Your intestinal tract has been inactive for a week or more, and the body is not prepared to take in and digest solid nourishment in an instant.

Breaking a fast is an art in itself. Don't hesitate to make a bit of a celebration out of it! After all, you've achieved something wonderful.

- Breakfast: You literally "break the fast" with a ripe, not too sour apple. Cut it in quarters and place on a plate. Then sit down to the feast and enjoy the fine apple aroma. Chew slowly and deliberately.
- Lunch: Eat the usual vegetable broth, but at this time add the solid vegetables, which should be pureed. You may eat a cracker or toast if you like.
- In the afternoon you can eat a low-fat yogurt.
- Supper: Have the soup with pureed vegetables once again.

After this first day of ending the fast, you can eat normally once again. "Normally" now means: not too much, not too fatty, and not too rich in calories. Get a calorie table and find out how many calories you generally consume in a day. Women should consume a daily ration of 1,500 to a maximum of 2,000 calories, and men from 2,000 to a maximum of 2,400 calories. These numbers apply to people who are moderately active.

When you stick to these limitations, you will maintain a steady weight and will remain slender. The Turbo-Protein Diet not only helps you rapidly lose excess pounds, but will stimulate better thyroid gland function. It might be a good idea to take 3 to 4 tablespoons of protein powder before your meals every once in a while, even after the diet is completed. This helps you to maintain your basal metabolism at a steady high level.

It is very easy to achieve an ideal weight that suits you— while maintaining good health in the process!

After the fast period, you might gain 2 to 5 pounds, which corresponds to the 1 or 2 quarts of water your body will retain in order to process solid foods again. This is no fat gain, this is a perfectly normal, healthy reaction of your body to prevent its dehydration.

COMMON QUESTIONS ABOUT
THE TURBO-PROTEIN DIET

What's so special about the protein drink?

In order to take advantage of the body's own metabolic processes so you can lose weight in a healthy way, the body must have a highly nutritional source of essential amino acids, even when it's being forced to fast. The required amount of protein is extremely large and cannot be provided with normal food, even with animal protein. Almased is a combination of soy protein, milk protein, and honey enzymes, and contains all the amino acids in their natural configuration (with a left twist), in the proportions required by the body. The body more easily recognizes these proteins and absorbs them immediately because they have been pre-fermented. The tasty powder is produced without any chemical additives and has not been pressure or heat treated, or denatured in any way. The average protein content per 100 grams of powder is approximately 53 percent, which is extremely high.

Who will profit the most from the Turbo-Protein Diet?

People who suffer from fatty metabolism diseases, high blood pressure, and high blood sugar up to levels including diabetes mellitus can all have great success with the Turbo-Protein

Diet. Falling blood sugar levels favor the elimination of disease-causing free radicals. The sports program simultaneously trains the insulin receptors in the muscles. If less medication is used to decrease the blood sugar, then fewer dosages of insulin are required. The stimulation of the metabolism causes a switch from the driving nature of the sympathetic nervous system, to the quieting effect of the parasympathetic nervous system, which in turn helps relax those who are overly tense. Blood pressure automatically drops, and medication can be spared.

WARNING!: In cases of serious metabolic illnesses, this diet may be carried out only under the auspices of a physician. But anyone can profit from this diet who wants to prevent suffering metabolic syndrome and desires to lose weight.

How often can you do the Turbo-Protein Diet?

After you have lost 10 or 20 pounds within two weeks, you should take a break from the diet for at least two or three weeks, depending on your metabolic condition and your exercise level. During this time, however, exercise a lot and do not overeat! Remember, women must eat 1,500 to 2,000 calories a day, and men, 2,000 to 2,400 calories a day. Afterwards you can begin again with the diet, in order to take off any remaining excess weight. For those who are extremely overweight, it is a good idea to fast for two weeks every three months, so that at the end of the year there is no chance that pants will pinch or skirts will be too tight. Otherwise there are no limitations for applying this diet.

After following the Turbo-Protein Diet, must I spend the rest of my life eating strictly low-calorie meals?

No! Heating up your metabolism with the protein drink is like a vaccination that needs only occasional boosters. Once your metabolism is properly revved up, you may eat normally. Once in a while take a few teaspoons of the protein powder in a drink, or perhaps mixed in yogurt or salad dressing. This is enough to keep the metabolism tuned up; everything in your body has been trained—even the thyroid gland function!

Can I work during this diet, or must I curb my activities?

While on the Turbo-Protein Diet your life can be perfectly normal, and you will be fully capable of handling your normal work load. You will sleep better, but often somewhat less, since your sleep will be more intense. Due to your body's switch over to the parasympathetic nervous system, you should try to approach everything a bit slower than usual, keeping your composure. After about the third day of fasting, when your body begins to burn up fat, you will experience the first sense of "having the wind at your back." Ketone bodies released during fat metabolism will give you a euphoric feeling, and it will seem like you are "floating through the fast cure." This turbo effect is strengthened by the endorphins released during sports. If, on the other hand, your mood becomes dark and you begin to feel depressed, it is likely that you are facing some inner conflict that is now coming out into the open. In this case you should see a therapist. Discordant feelings cannot be attributed to the Turbo-Protein Diet itself. Quite the contrary, it very well may help you approach life with increased ease and enjoyment.

Can a fasting crisis occur?

Except in the above-mentioned case, which must be seen in another context, you will not experience any fasting crisis during the Turbo-Protein Diet. The old diet motto of perseverance, "Grin and bear it!" is nothing less than the worst sort of contempt for vital physiological laws. Fasting crises are basically massive stress symptoms, which can occur during conventional diets and include weakness (feeling faint), bad sleep, sweat outbursts, weak circulation, sexual disinterest, headaches, attacks of hunger, and so forth.

Do bodily functions change during the fast?
Does one have to reckon with limitations?

No, just the opposite is true; in fact, your sex life can become more intense. In addition to the powerful stimulation of the thyroid gland, it seems that the production of sex hormones also clearly increases. Many of my patients joyfully report this pleasant side effect. Another slight change is that your body eliminates more while you are on this diet,. The urine can smell stronger, and increased sweating is also sometimes observed. Both effects are very favorable signs that an intensive and effective purifying process is taking place in the body.

Is old age an obstacle to trying the protein diet?

No, quite the contrary. Especially in old age, a slender figure and consuming highly nourishing, easily digestible protein is of great importance. After about the age of fifty, the absorption capacity of the gastrointestinal tract wanes considerably. Deficits develop, especially in the absorption and conversion of protein; as a result, the muscles start to shrink, the skin becomes slack, glandular functions decline, sexuality tends to wane, and the bones become brittle. All these symptoms of age can be combated with the help of the Turbo-Protein Diet. Taking part in a little bit of sports, appropriate for your abilities, is also beneficial.

Why does one burn up so much fat in this diet, and how does that work?

Eighty percent of the people on earth need no more than about 2,400 calories a day. While on this diet, the body is provided with a daily ration of only about 400 calories, creating a deficit of some 2,000 calories. Since the entire metabolic engine is revved up by the soy milk mixture, the burning process is increased by about 30 to 40 percent. On top of that, engaging in sports further enhances the engine's power, so that there is at least a 50 percent increase in the basal metabolism.

During the fast, the body's need for energy is—the 2,000 calorie deficit for normal metabolism, plus another 1,000 calories for the high-rev state created by the diet; therefore, 3,000 calories per day are required by your body. Since these calories are suddenly not available to the (properly fasting) organism, the body gets them out of its fat reserves. One pound of fat provides 2,750 calories of energy, so the body will burn as much as just over a pound of fat every day!

Therefore it is not surprising that 13 to 18 pounds of fat can be metabolized in only two weeks.

What enduring successes can be expected with the Turbo-Protein Diet?

My own studies of patients found a statistically significant success rate of losing weight, of forming the thyroid hormone T_4, and of increasing conversion of T_4 into T_3. Thyroid activity data revealed the vigorous stimulation of the metabolism. All told, men and women made equally good showings.

REFERENCES

Bässler, K.H.: "The role of carbohydrates in healthy nutrition — the role of sugar." Lecture at a continuing education seminar hosted by the Association of General Practitioners and Family Doctors of Germany (BPA), Landesverband Hamburg e.V., Hamburg, Germany, September 22, 1993

Bayer, W. et al.: *The Influence of Antioxidantly Effective Vitamins on the Parameters of the Cellular Immune System.* VitaMinSpur 5, 1990

German Society for Nutrition: *Recommendations for Nutritional Intake.* Umschau-Verlag, 5. Revision, Frankfurt, Germany, 1991

Frankel, E.N. et al.: *Inhibition of oxidation of human low-density lipoprotein by phenolic substances in red wine.* Lancet 341, 1993

Friedman J.M. Obesity. *Brown fat and yellow mice.* Nature 366, 1993

Leibel R.L. Bahary N. Friedman J.M.: *Strategies for the molecular genetic analysis of obesity in humans.* Crit-Rev-Food-Sci-Nutr. 1993

Fürst, P.: *Antioxidant Power of Nutrition — "non-nutritive" Substances.* Institute for Biological Chemistry and Nutritional Sciences at the University Stuttgart-Hohenheim. Lecture in Königswinter, Germany on April 9, 1994

Fumeron, F. et al.: *Lowering of HD_2-cholesterol and lipoprotein A-I particle levels bz increasing the ratio of polyunsaturated to saturated fatty acids.* AmJClinNutr 53, 1991

Gey, K.F.: *The antioxidant hypothesis of cardiovascular disease:*

epidemiology and mechanisms. Biochem Soc Trans 18, 1990

Grossklaus, R.: *The importance of sweetners in diets for weight control.* Ernährungsforschung 38, 1993

Grunert, S.C.: *Food and Emotions. The self-regulation of emotions through eating behavior.* Beltz Psychologie Verlags-Union, Weinheim, Germany, 1993

Grussendorf M.: *Metabolism of the thyroid hormones. Research on healthy and heavily diseased organisms.* G. Thieme Verlag, Stuttgart, 1988

Gertog, M.G. et al.: *Dietary antioxidant flavonoids and risk of coronarz heart disease: The Zutphen Elderly Study.* Lancet 342, 1993

Klever, U.: *Klever's calory-joule-compass 1995/96.* Gräfe und Unzer Verlag, München 1995

Kübler, W.: *Nutritional Problems.* Magazine of R.P. Scherer GmbH company, Eberbach/Baden, 1986

Kübler, W. et al.: *Food and Nutrition Intake of Adults in the Federal Republic of Germany.* VERA-Schriftenreihe Vol. III. Wissenschaftlicher Fachverlag Dr. Fleck, Niederkleen, 1992

Münzing-Ruef, I.: *Schedule for healthy nutrition.* Wilhelm Heyne Verlag, München, 1991

Stunkard, A.J. and T.A. Waaden: *Obesity Theory and Therapy.* Raven Press, New York, 1993

Truswell, A.S.: *Food carbohydrates and plasma lipids — an update.* American Journal of Clinical Nutrition (Supplement) 59, 1994

World Health Organization: *Diet, nutrition and the prevention of chronic diseases.* Report of a WHO Study Group. Technical Report Series 797, WHO, Geneva, 1990

The author's own study:
Increased basal metabolic rate by stimulation of the T_4/T_3-neo-genesis by means of a specific dynamic amino acid preparation: Bio. Med. (2): 1996: 75-78.

About the Author

Dieter Markert attended medical school in Frankfurt, Germany and continued his education and specialization in anesthesiology, resuscitation, and general pain therapy. He currently maintains a general practice with an emphasis on naturopathic pain therapy and scientific research.

Dr. Markert and a large number of his patients have personally tested this diet program with remarkable success.

A LETTER TO THE READER

Dear Reader:

In 1992, scientists received a Nobel award for discovering the effects of proteins in combination with enzymes. Enzymes enable your body to digest nutritional proteins, or better: they help your body transform nutritional proteins into new cells.

We at ALMASED have put this discovery to use for you by manufacturing a meal replacement formula which gives your body a lot of the nutritional elements that it is underfed with, mostly proteins and enzymes. It contains a large amount of soy protein, the best plant protein.* Skim milk yogurt provides additional protein, while raw honey supplies the necessary enzymes. All ingredients are organic materials, and the right combination makes it easy on your body to completely digest them all.

Rheumatism, gout, circulatory disturbances, diabetes, lack of drive, early loss of vitality, being overweight etc. are often the indications of bad eating habits and of a bad metabolism. A lot of people have problems with their digestive system like stomach and liver which causes their entire metabolism to malfunction.

Having read *The Turbo Protein Diet* you are about to join thousands of successful dieters. Please remember: Weight loss is hard work for your body. If you don't supplement your diet with a product like ALMASED, you may experience deficiency symptoms, muscle decrease and/or slow down of your metabolism. ALMASED provides your body with essential parts to create new cells. It will keep you feeling full for several hours and reduce your appetite. ALMASED keeps your metabolism going, so fat really burns off while regulating your insulin to avoid future weight gain (the "yo-yo effect"). In other words: You feel great as fat goes.

More and more people take ALMASED worldwide. ALMASED can be mixed in many drinks and foods. Three teaspoons of ALMASED three times daily provide you with energy, power and vitality. It fills, reduces your appetite and stimulates your metabolism.

If you have any questions about this unique new product or would like to take advantage of our incredible introductory offer, call nationwide toll free 1-877-ALMASED (1-877-256-2733).*

Yours sincerely,
Andre Trouille
President ALMASED USA, Inc.

* People allergic to soy should check with their doctor before using this product.